THE NEW LIFE LIBRARY

INSTANT
AROMATHERAPY

FOR STRESS RELIEF

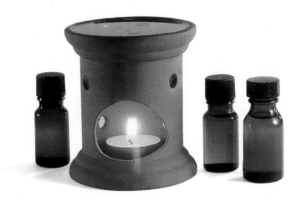

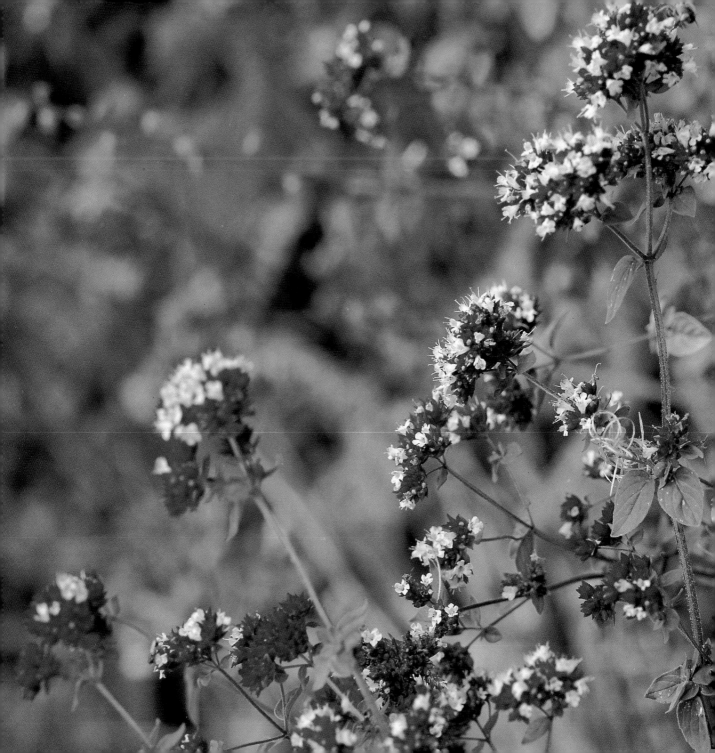

THE NEW LIFE LIBRARY

INSTANT AROMATHERAPY

FOR STRESS RELIEF

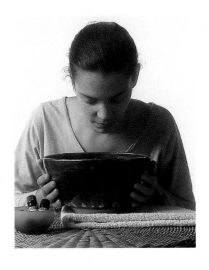

SIMPLE

TENSION

TREATMENTS

AND

RELAXATION

RECIPES

MARK EVANS

LORENZ BOOKS

LONDON • NEW YORK • SYDNEY • BATH

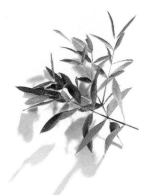
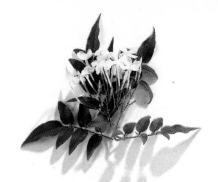

First published in 1996 by Lorenz Books

© 1996 Anness Publishing Limited

Lorenz Books is an imprint of
Anness Publishing Limited
Boundary Row Studios
1 Boundary Row
London SE1 8HP

This edition distributed in Canada by Raincoast Books Distribution Limited.

ISBN 1 85976 289 2

A CIP catalogue record is available from the British Library

Publisher: Joanna Lorenz
Editor: Fiona Eaton
Designer: Bobbie Colgate Stone
Photographer: Don Last

Printed in China

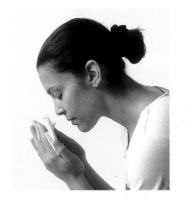

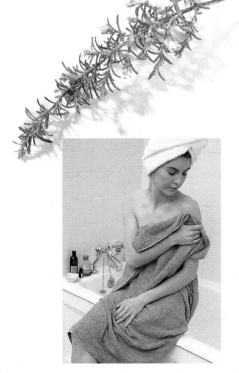

CONTENTS

AROMATHERAPY — AN ANCIENT ART

DO YOU HAVE A FAVOURITE SCENT, one that evokes memories of wonderful times and places? The power of the sense of smell to arouse an instant emotional reaction confirms its ability to have an immediate effect on our systems; smell is probably the most underrated of the senses, yet it has the most subtle significance in our lives. Most of our pleasure from foods relies on their aroma; the initial attraction (or otherwise!) of other people probably depends on their scent as much as anything else.

Moods can be enhanced or changed with the use of scents; some of the most concentrated aromas are found within the plant kingdom. Aromatic plants contain essential oils that have been used for centuries to relax, sedate, refresh or stimulate according to need.

How do these substances work? Airborne aromatic molecules are detected by the brain's olfactory centre via the nostrils, and produce an immediate emotional or instinctive response from the limbic system within the brain. Aromatic essential oils can have significant physiological and pharmacological effects as well as affecting moods. Aromatic molecules may enter the lungs and become absorbed into the bloodstream which can carry them to all parts of the body. When used on the skin, aromatic compounds are also absorbed directly into the bloodstream in the same way.

Each aromatic oil has its own individual combination of constituents; these in turn can interact with your body's chemistry to have specific therapeutic effects. Particular aromatic compounds will affect certain organs; for example, when garlic is eaten, it is

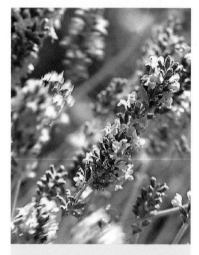

Essential oils are natural, volatile substances that evaporate readily, releasing their aroma into the air, as happens, for example, when someone brushes against an aromatic plant. Essential oils are produced by specialized glands present in some plants.

Right: One of the most versatile, relaxing and healing oils is lavender.

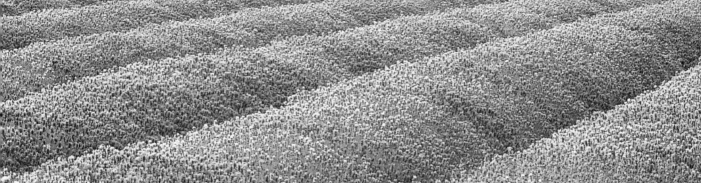

excreted 99 per cent via the lungs, hence its therapeutic benefits on respiratory infections (and also why it causes smelly breath).

The origins and development of our knowledge of aromatic oils coincide with the history of mankind; people have been using scented products since time began. Ancient written records, whether they be the Vedic manuscripts from India dating back some 3,000 years, Egyptian papyri from 1500 BC or biblical stories of the Jewish exodus from Egypt about 300 years later, all describe the widespread use of aromatic oils. Many were used not only in religious ceremonies and rituals but also in massage, in the bath and for scenting the hair and body.

While the Egyptians, Greeks and Romans made lavish use of aromatic preparations, it has been thought that they did not know how to distil the pure essential oils from plants. This is generally credited to the Arabic physicians of the tenth century AD; however, archaeological evidence from the Indus valley in the foothills of the Himalayas indicates that distillation may have been known 5,000 years ago. Certainly, the Arabic use of concentrated, distilled oils – famed in the West as the "perfumes of Arabia" – led to a renaissance in the usage of aromatic plants.

As distillation was taken up in the West, many more oils were extracted. There was also a gradual separation of perfumery and more medical applications; the latter led into synthetic chemistry, and a loss of the sense of the psychological aspects of aroma. Ironically, it was from the perfumery industry that much of the impetus came for the development of aromatherapy; indeed the very name was coined by a perfumer.

In the early years of the twentieth century, a French chemist René-Maurice Gattefosse was working in the laboratory of his family's perfumery business, when he

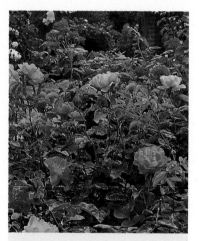

When you breathe in an aroma, you get an instant emotional reaction; this may be related to past experiences, recalling a memory associated with the smell, or just instinctive pleasure or dislike. Some oils are sedating, others highly uplifting, but these qualities will be altered by your psychological reactions.

burnt his hand and lower arm badly. He plunged his hand into the nearest liquid, which was a jar of lavender oil, and discovered that this very quickly eased the pain, prevented scarring and promoted rapid healing. Gattefosse then began to investigate the therapeutic properties of essential oils, discovering that they were often more effective than isolated or synthetic compounds. In 1928 he used the term aromatherapy to describe the use of aromatic oils for treating physical or emotional problems.

Another significant person in the development of aromatherapy was Dr Jean Valnet. He used essential oils to treat a number of conditions, ranging from his wartime experience treating infections and diseases to the use of aromatherapy for people suffering from psychiatric disorders. This kind of work started to bridge the gap again between the medical/physical properties and emotional effects of aromatic oils.

Aromatherapists today may use specific essential oils for their physiological effects, but there is no reason why these may not be used for their relaxing properties, if used carefully. Essential oils are often produced by plants as part of their defences against predators, and they should always be treated with respect. In this book the focus is on their role in stress reduction.

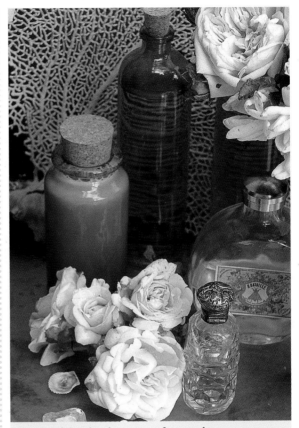

Much of the development of aromatherapy came from the perfumery industry, initially with the distillation of essential oils and then with the creative blending of aromatic oils to make harmonious scents. The concept of combining oils is also relevant to aromatherapy, since the effects of individual oils can be magnified in combination. A balanced scent from a blend is likely to be more enjoyable and have a greater therapeutic effect.

USING AND PREPARING OILS

AROMATIC ESSENTIAL OILS may be used in a number of ways to maintain and restore health, and to improve the quality of life with their scents. Essential oils are concentrated substances and as such they need to be diluted for safety and optimum effect. Treat them with care and respect – and allow them to treat you!

Essential oils are liable to deteriorate through the action of sunlight, so should be stored in a cool, dark place. They are sold in dark glass dropper bottles which protect the oils from the light and help with measuring. Only blend a small quantity of oils at a time to prevent the mixture deteriorating.

Many companies now sell essential oils; make sure that they are pure and of a high quality (you get what you pay for in general). If possible, try to smell a sample bottle of the oil you are buying in a shop – does it have a clean, non-synthetic odour with just one aromatic "note", or can you detect more than one scent? The latter may mean the oil is not so pure or fresh. Also beware of very cheap oils; what may seem to be a bargain may be of very little value for aromatherapy purposes and may even cause headaches or other reactions if used in excess.

For using essential oils at home, it can be helpful to have a little equipment. For vaporizing oils into the atmosphere, a burner is an easy option; simmering potpourri in a bowl with a candle underneath is another more unusual way to make a room fragrant, while a long-term scent, although fainter, can be achieved with a bowl of dry potpourri.

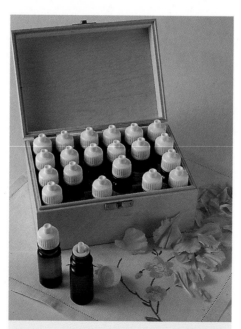

Keep essential oils in dark glass dropper bottles, out of the light to prevent deterioration by sunlight.

Right: Essential oils can be used in a burner or added to potpourri.

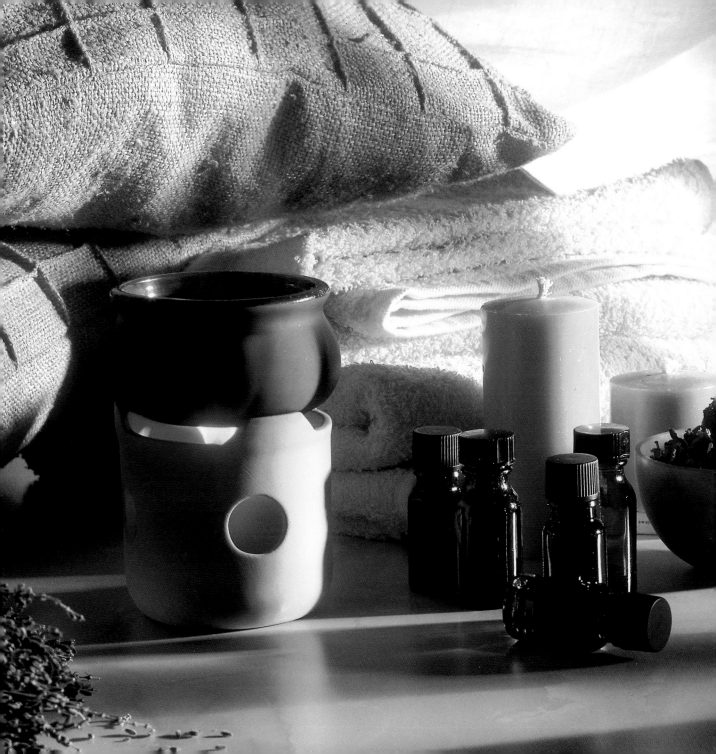

MASSAGE

Massage is a wonderful way to use essential oils, suitably diluted in a good base oil, for your partner or family. Use soft, thick towels to cover areas of the body you are not massaging, and make sure that the room is warm, perhaps with an additional portable heater.

Suitable base oils include sweet almond oil (probably the most versatile and useful), grapeseed, safflower, soya (a bit thicker and stickier), coconut and even sunflower. For very dry skins, a small amount of jojoba, avocado or wheatgerm oils (except in cases of wheat allergy) may be added. Essential oils may be blended at a dilution of 1 per cent, or one drop per 5 ml (1 tsp) of base oil; this may sometimes be increased to 2 per cent, but take care that no skin reactions occur with any oil.

CAUTION:
If someone has sensitive skin or suffers from allergies, then try massaging with just one drop of essential oil per 20 ml (4 tsp) of base oil at first to test for any reaction (rare). Seek medical advice before massaging a pregnant woman.

Right: One of the nicest ways of using aromatic essential oils is diluted in a base massage oil.

MIXING ESSENTIAL OILS FOR MASSAGE

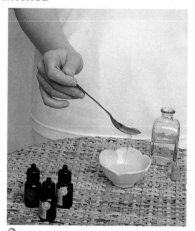

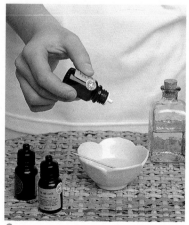

1 Before you begin, wash and dry your hands and make sure that all the utensils are clean and dry. Measure out about 10 ml (2 tsp) of your chosen vegetable oil.

2 Pour the vegetable oil into the blending bowl.

3 Add the essential oil, one drop at a time. Mix gently with a clean, dry cocktail stick or toothpick.

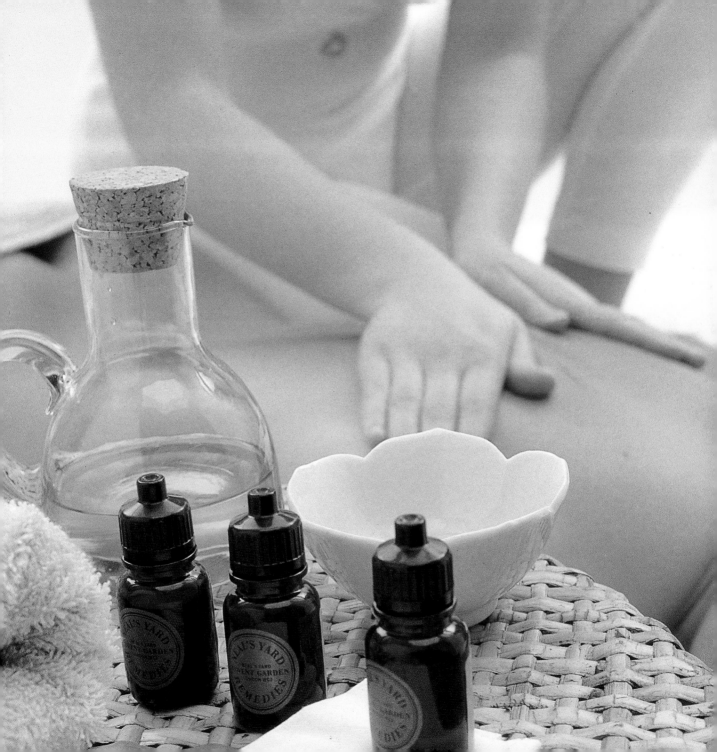

BATHS

Imagine soaking in a hot bath, enveloped in a delicious scent of exotic flowers, feeling all the day's tensions drop away . . . well, that can be a reality with aromatherapy. The oils seem to capture the essence of the plant, and can effortlessly transport you to pine-scented forests, refreshing orange groves or oriental spice markets.

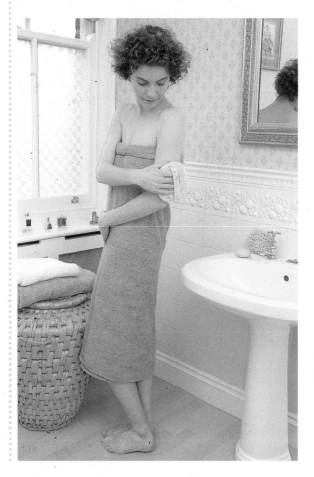

When using oils in the bath, pour in 5 drops just before you get in. The oils form a thin film on the surface of the water and this, aided by the warmth of the water, will be partly absorbed by your skin while you breathe in the scent, producing an immediate psychological and physiological effect.

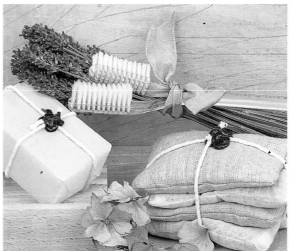

Left: Rubbing the body with a loofah increases the effectiveness of an aromatherapy bath. Above: Lavender has long been associated with bathing. Right: Essential oil in a burner will fragrance a room.

MORNING BATH

For a refreshing, uplifting bath in the mornings try a blend of 3 drops bergamot and 2 drops geranium essential oils.

EVENING BATH

To relax and unwind after a long day, make a blend of 3 drops lavender and 2 drops ylang ylang to add to your bath.

BATH FOR ACHING MUSCLES

For tired, tense muscles, soak in a bath to which you have added 3 drops marjoram and 2 drops chamomile essential oils.

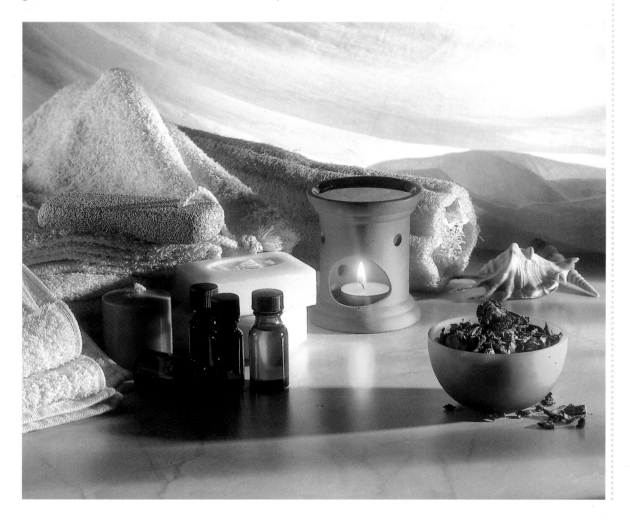

HAND AND FOOTBATHS

A quick way to use essential oils is to make a hand or footbath; two-thirds fill a large bowl with hot water and add 3–4 drops of oil. Circulation to our extremities is affected by tension and stress, among other things, and the warmth of the water itself helps the blood vessels to dilate. This can be very helpful in treating conditions such as tension headaches and migraines, when the blood vessels in the head are frequently engorged with blood. If you regularly suffer from these problems, try a foot or handbath at the first signs of a headache and see if you can drain away the excess stress.

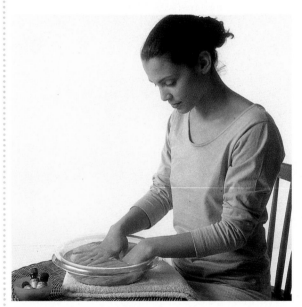

CIRCULATION
For poor circulation and tense, cold extremities, add 2 drops lavender and 2 drops marjoram oils.

ACHING MUSCLES: OVER-EXERTION
For tension and stiffness, perhaps from overuse, try a blend of 2 drops rosemary and 2 drops pine.

EXCESS HEAT: WHEN HOT AND BOTHERED
For hot, aching feet or hands, use a mixture of 2 drops peppermint and 2 drops lemon.

Left: Handbaths are a simple way of enjoying the benefits of essential oils. Below: Peppermint is cooling and counteracts tiredness. The essential oil is ideal for using in a refreshing footbath.

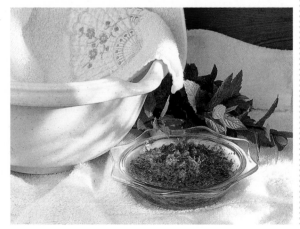

STEAM INHALATIONS

Colds and sinus problems may cause congestion, but we can also feel blocked up and unable to breathe freely through tension. Using a steam inhalation warms and moistens the membranes, and the use of essential oils helps to open and relax the airways. Just boil a kettle, pour the water into a bowl, add the oils and inhale deeply.

NASAL CONGESTION

For a stuffed-up feeling, maybe combined with tiredness, try using 3 drops eucalyptus and 2 drops peppermint in a bowl of steaming water.

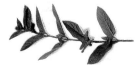

TIGHT, TENSE CHEST

For tension causing poor breathing, relax the airways with 4 drops lavender and 3 drops frankincense.

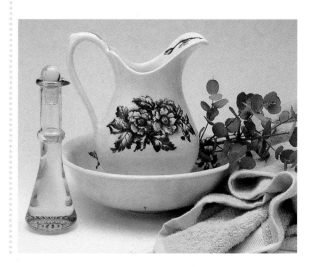

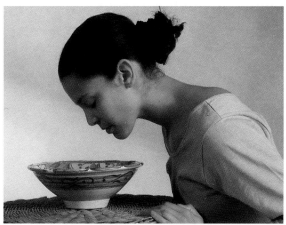

Above: For respiratory complaints in particular, steam inhalations are very helpful. Use a total of 10 drops for a strong medicinal effect, in cases of colds and chestiness, or just 5 drops for a gentler relaxing effect on the airways. Left: Eucalyptus is particularly effective at clearing the chest and nose.

CAUTION:
If you have high blood pressure or asthma seek medical advice before using steam, and in any case do not overdo an inhalation.

SCENTED ROOMS

Aromatherapy has many applications in the home or office including the creation
of an aromatic environment which has wide-ranging beneficial effects.

POTPOURRI

It is possible to scent a room by making a simmering
potpourri. Place a mixture of scented flowers and
leaves (without any fixatives or additives) in a bowl of
water and heat gently from below – a candle may well
be sufficient. Unlike dry potpourri, the simmering
variety does not last for long but gives off a much
stronger aroma at the time. Try making your own
blends, using your nose to achieve the aroma you
desire; add about 1 cupful of dried material to 1.2
litres (2 pints) of water.

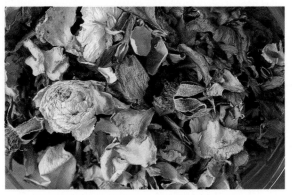

Potpourri gives a long-lasting fragrance to the air.

For a sleep-enhancing simmering potpourri
blend try using ½ cup lime flowers, ¼ cup
chamomile flowers, 1 tbsp sweet marjoram and 1 tbsp
lavender flowers. For a more refreshing, uplifting
blend try mixing together ½ cup lemon verbena
leaves, ¼ cup jasmine flowers, 2 tbsp lemon peel and
1 tsp coriander seeds.

ESSENTIAL OIL BURNERS

Most oils lend themselves to use in a burner. The
basic principle is very simple: a small dish to hold a
few drops of essential oil, with some type of gentle
heat underneath, often in the form of a candle. The
heat needs to be fairly low, in order to allow slow
evaporation of the oil and a longer-lasting scent.

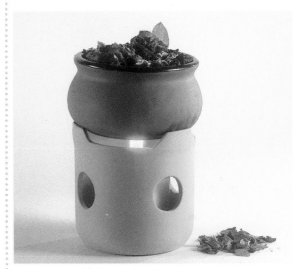

Special potpourri burners are now widely available.

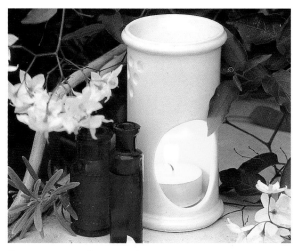

Burners can make attractive room ornaments.

If you want to fumigate a room, then try adding 3–4 drops of oils such as pine, eucalyptus or juniper to a burner. To help you keep alert, then a couple of drops of peppermint or rosemary may be appropriate, while 2–3 drops of ylang ylang or lavender will help you to wind down at the end of the day.

BOWL OF HOT WATER

Adding a couple of drops of an essential oil to a bowl of hot water can be a pleasant way to give fragrance to a room or office, especially if the atmosphere is dry as a result of central heating. Choose an attractive bowl and place it out of reach of children. Use an oil that you really like, as its scent will linger for some time.

For mornings, one of the fresh aromas such as bergamot, mandarin or lemon would be uplifting. Later in the day you may wish to use a floral essence, such as rose or jasmine, which have calming effects.

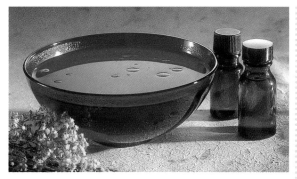

A few drops of oil in hot water will scent a room.

OTHER SCENTED PRODUCTS

Essential oils are quite often included in items such as scented candles, incense sticks or cones, and other aromatic products. It is important to check that natural essential oils have been used to scent these products before you buy them; synthetic perfumes may have a similar scent but they will not have the beneficial therapeutic properties of natural plant extracts.

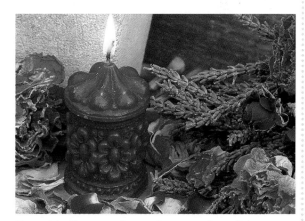

Essential oils are used to make scented candles.

COMPRESSES

Hot or cold compresses are excellent ways to use oils for problems such as sprains and muscular aches. To make a cold compress, pour cold water over some ice in a bowl, add essential oils and soak a pad in the water before placing over the affected area and binding firmly in place. For a hot compress, have the water as hot as you can comfortably bear and pour into a bowl, add oils and use as above. Use 3–4 drops of essential oils in an average sized cereal bowl.

Cold compresses are suitable for use on acute injuries such as a strain or sprain, with swelling or bruising. For older injuries, with no swelling or inflammation, for chronic muscle aches such as backache and menstrual pain, and for arthritic or rheumatic pain, a hot compress may be more useful.

The ideal essential oil for a cold compress is lavender, and this can be very useful in many first aid situations. Use 4 drops to a bowl of iced water. Keep the pad on firmly for at least 20 minutes, preferably with the affected limb raised if there is any swelling.

For muscular aches and pains, try using 2 drops of both rosemary and marjoram in a bowl of hot water. Apply the compress for 30 minutes.

CAUTION:
For any major injury always seek medical advice or treatment.

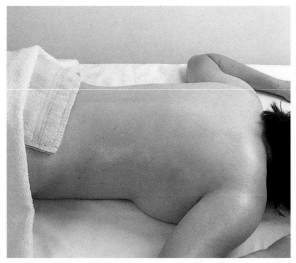

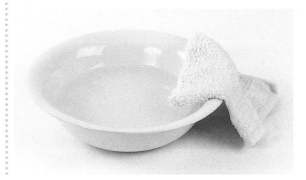

Left: Aromatherapy oils can be added to warm water to make a soothing compress. Above: Compresses can stimulate circulation and reduce inflammation.

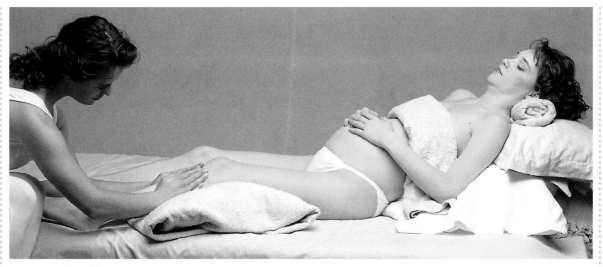

Gentle massage during pregnancy can be very relaxing. However, you should always seek medical advice first.

CAUTION:

Essential oils are wonderful natural remedies for a variety of problems, and their aromatic effects can enhance mood, release tensions and reduce stress. But they are highly concentrated substances and must be used with caution. Follow the advice given below and if in any doubt seek a medical opinion before using them.

• Never take essential oils internally, unless professionally prescribed.

• Always use essential oils diluted – normally 1 per cent for massage; just 5 drops in a bath or for a steam inhalation.

• Do not use the same oils for too long, follow the "1–2 rule"; use one or two oils together, for not more than one or two weeks at any one time.

• Do not use oils in pregnancy, without getting professional advice; some oils, such as basil, clary sage, juniper, marjoram and sage, are contra-indicated at this time.

• For anyone who has any skin problems, dilute the oils even more and if any skin irritation occurs stop using them immediately. A few essential oils, such as bergamot, make the skin more sensitive to sunlight, so should be used with caution in hot, sunny weather.

• Be extra careful with anyone who has asthma or epilepsy, and if anyone experiences a reaction, then stop using the oil.

SELF-MASSAGE

Give yourself a real treat with these simple self-massage techniques. Choose an appropriate blend of essential oils from the pages of this book, and add at 1 per cent to a base oil such as sweet almond. Oil your hands before spreading it on to your skin, and feel your tension knots unwind!

THE FACE

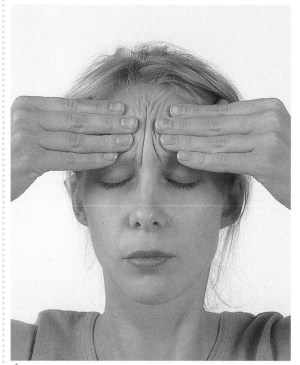 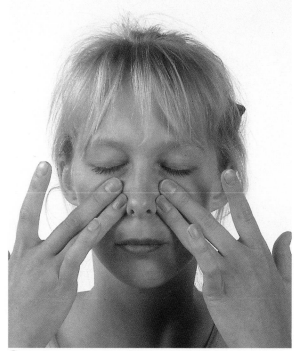

1 Use small, slow circling movements with the fingers, working steadily from the forehead down around the temples and over the cheeks. Use firm pressure and work slowly to ease tensions out of all the facial muscles.

2 Work across the cheeks and along each side of the nose, then move out to the jaw line where a lot of tension is held. Try not to pull downwards on the skin – let the circling movements help to smooth the stresses away and gently lift the face as you work.

THE HANDS

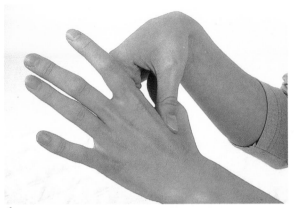

1 Help to reduce tension in the hands by firmly squeezing between each finger with the thumb and fingers of the other hand, rolling the flesh a little to give a kneading effect.

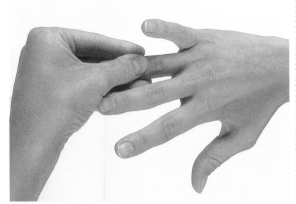

2 Squeeze and gently stretch each finger in turn, working from the hand out to the fingertip.

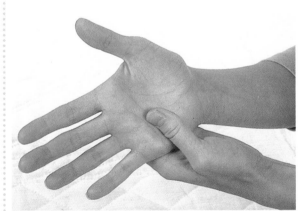

3 With a firm movement, knead the palm with the thumb of your other hand, making strong circular strokes. This squeezes and stretches taut, contracted muscles, and should be a fairly deep action.

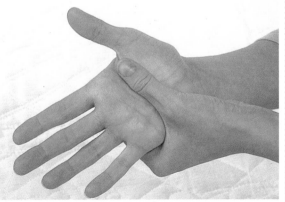

4 Work steadily over the palm, maintaining a firm pressure. Repeat these movements on the other hand.

THE ARMS

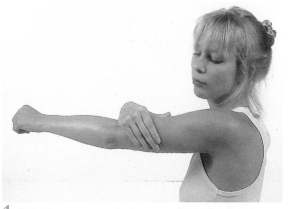 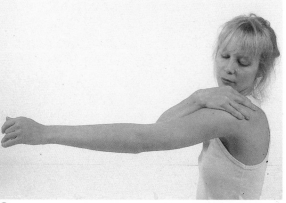

1 Grip your outstretched arm at the wrist, between the thumb and fingers of the other hand and squeeze firmly. Repeat, moving up the arm.

2 Continue this kneading movement all the way up the arm to the shoulder. You can perform this stroke two or three times, working upwards each time, then switch arms and repeat.

THE SHOULDERS

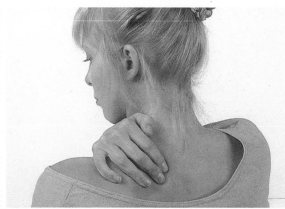 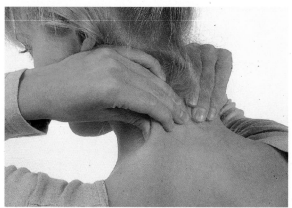

1 Firmly grip your shoulder and use a squeezing motion to loosen the tension, moving along the shoulder several times. Repeat on the other side.

2 Work up as far as the base of the skull squeezing the neck muscles with your fingertips, and down again.

THE LEGS

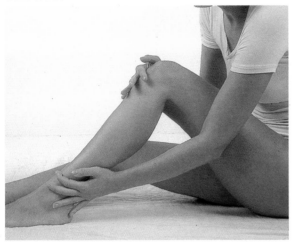 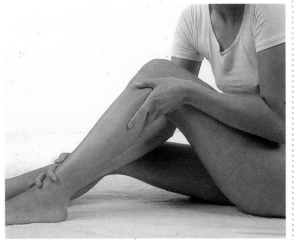

1 Sit with one leg bent, so that you can comfortably reach down as far as the ankle.

2 With steady, fairly firm movements sweep up the leg from ankle to knee, using alternate hands. This movement helps to move venous blood back toward the heart as well as working on the calf muscles. If you suffer from aching legs, then do a little sweeping movement on the upper leg first, from knee to hip, in the same way, to aid circulation. Repeat the movements on the other leg.

THE FEET

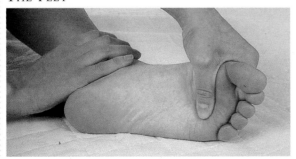

◀ Sit so that you can comfortably reach a foot, and with quite a firm grip use small circular strokes all over the sole with your thumb. Pay special attention to the arch of the foot, stretching along the line of the arch with your thumb. Change or adjust your position and repeat on the other foot.

MASSAGE WITH A PARTNER

One of the best ways to take away stress and tension from your partner is to use massage. The effects of the following simple massage movements can be greatly enhanced by adding essential oils, at 1 per cent dilution, to the base oil. Remember, when using essential oils in massage you are sharing the fragrance and therapeutic effect, so choose a blend that you both like.

Prepare the massage space beforehand, making sure it is warm and comfortable. Make sure that your partner is lying comfortably: use cushions or pillows for support if necessary, and cover with towels if needed to keep warm. Warm the oil in your hands before applying to the skin and then let your fingers get to work.

THE BACK

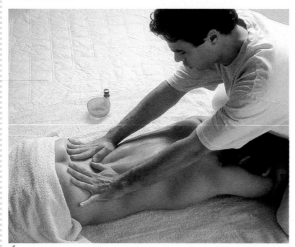

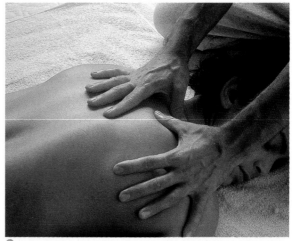

1 Sit or kneel at the head end, and place your hands on either side of the spine, on the line of muscles that run down the back. With a steady gliding motion move down the back as far as the pelvis, if you can reach comfortably; take your hands further out to the side and glide back up to the shoulders, before repeating this stroke. Move slowly, without stopping.

2 For shoulder tensions and stiffness, use your thumbs to work in small, deeper circles around the shoulder blade. Adjust the pressure to suit your partner – do not inflict discomfort! Repeat the circling movement around each shoulder in turn.

THE FACE AND HEAD

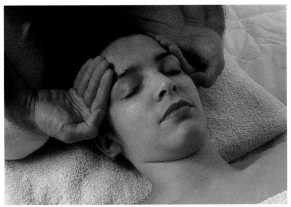

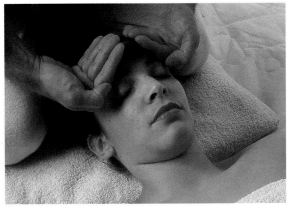

1 Smooth across the forehead with the back of your hands. Start the stroking motion at the centre of the forehead and move towards the temples.

2 These movements can often ease a headache, especially at an early stage, and are very calming.

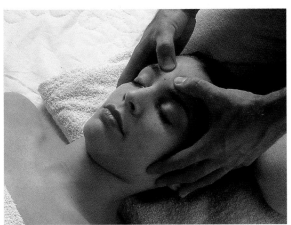

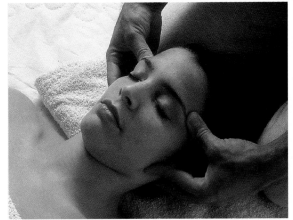

3 Using your thumbs or fingers, work steadily over the forehead in small circles, moving out over the temples to ease tight, tense muscles.

4 You can continue this movement down the temples to the jaw line for an even greater relaxing effect. Use fairly firm pressure, squeezing the skin with each circle rather than just moving over the top of the skin.

THE ARMS

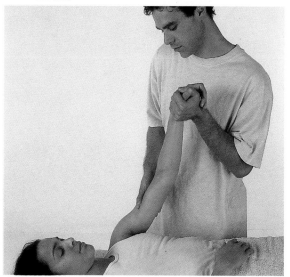

1 Support your partner's arm, raising it into the air and steadily squeeze down the whole length of the arm with your thumb and fingers to encourage blood and lymph flow back towards the heart.

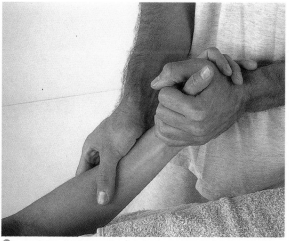

2 Let the upper arm rest on the floor, then work on the forearm with firm stroking movements from the wrist to the elbow – you may need to swap your hands in order to work around each side of the arm.

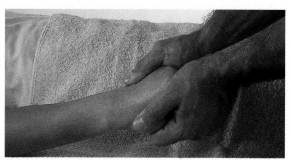

3 To help relieve tension from your partner's hands, hold a hand, palm down, in your hands and apply a steady stretching motion across the back of the hand.

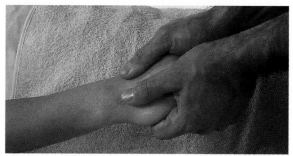

4 Repeat this stretch a few times, with a firm but comfortable pressure on the hand. Repeat all these movements on the other arm and hand.

THE FEET

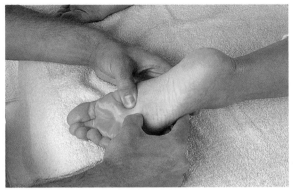

1 Use your thumbs to press firmly in small circles all over the sole. Keep the movements slow and quite deep, and finish with long lines running from the toes to the heel to stretch along the arch. Repeat on the other foot.

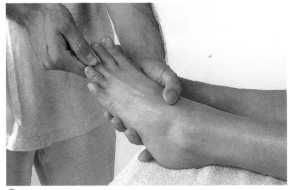

2 Hold one of the toes and give a squeeze and pulling action. Repeat for all the toes.

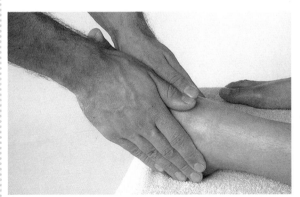

3 Smooth all the way up and down the upper side of the foot with both hands.

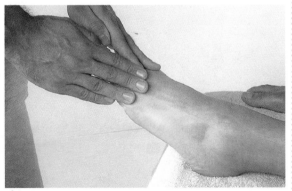

4 Extend the smooth stroking motion from the ankle all the way to the toes. Return to the center and smooth back up the foot. Repeat on the other foot.

THE OILS

ESSENTIAL OILS MAY BE EXTRACTED from exotic plants such as sandalwood or ylang ylang, or from more common plants like lavender and chamomile, but each one has its own characteristics and properties. Try to get used to a few oils at first, understand their effects, and enjoy their fragrance!

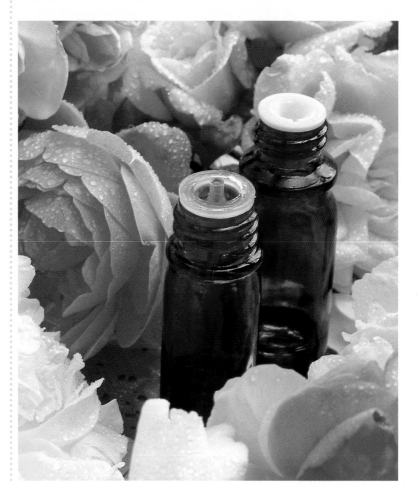

Left: Essential oils are concentrated substances; while the skin of citrus fruits such as lemon or orange may yield a fair amount of oil, flowers such as roses only contain tiny amounts of the precious essence – about 5,000 roses may be needed to obtain 5 ml (1 tsp) of pure essential oil. This concentration emphasizes the importance of only using drop doses of the oils, in a suitable dilution, as a little goes a long way.

Right: Oils are extracted from many different parts of plants. Each contains powerful healing properties, to be enjoyed but also respected. Nature provides an abundance of therapeutic compounds to help us regain health and vitality.

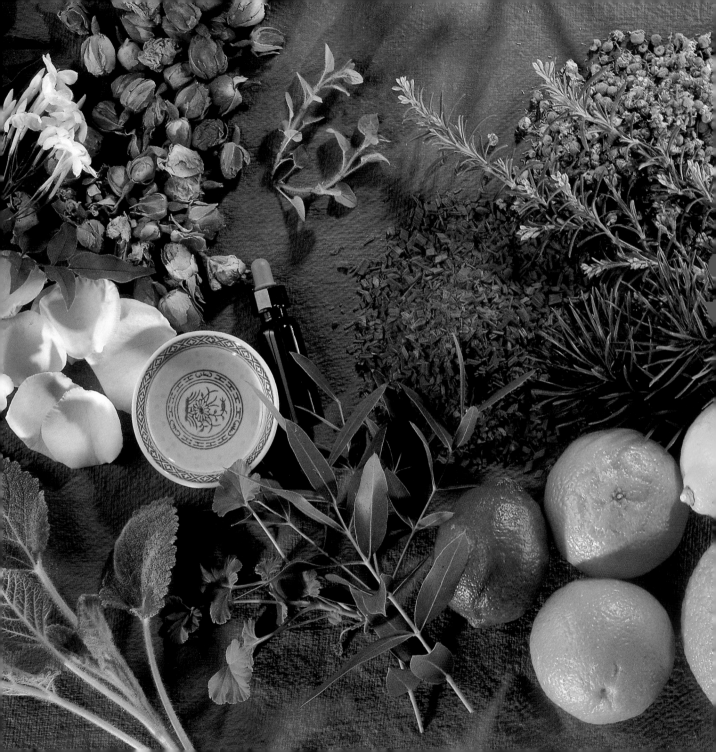

SANDALWOOD (*SANTALUM ALBUM*)

Probably the oldest perfume in history, known to have been used for over 4,000 years. Sandalwood has a heavy scent, and often appeals to men as much as to women. It has a relaxing, antidepressant effect on the nervous system, and where depression causes sexual problems, sandalwood can be a genuine aphrodisiac.

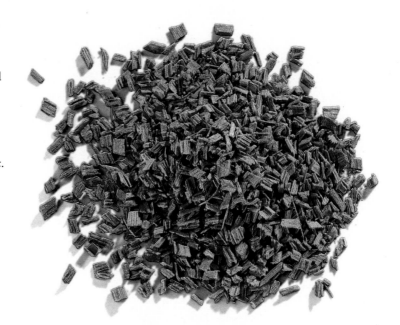

CHAMOMILE (*MATRICARIA RECUTITA* [German] OR *CHAMAEMELUM NOBILE* [Roman])

Roman and German chamomile are both used to obtain essential oils with very similar properties. Chamomile is relaxing and antispasmodic, helping to relieve tension headaches, nervous digestive problems or insomnia, for instance.

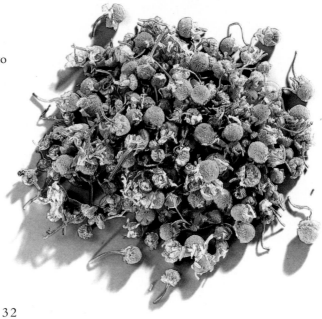

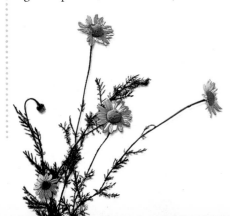

BENZOIN (*STYRAX BENZOIN*)

This Asiatic tree produces a gum which is usually dissolved in a solvent to produce the "oil". It has a wonderful fragrance of vanilla, and is widely used in inhalation mixtures. It relaxes the airways and can be used whenever tension leads to a tight chest or restricted breathing.

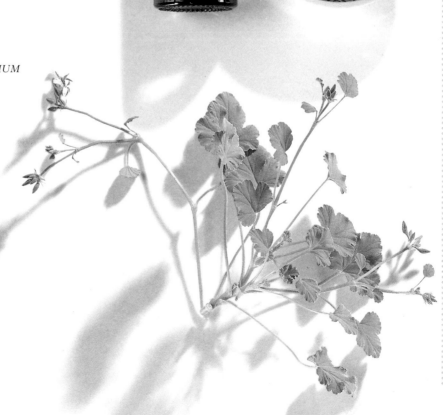

GERANIUM (*PELARGONIUM GRAVEOLENS*)

The rose-scented geranium has very useful properties, not least being its ability to bring a blend together, to make a more harmonious scent. Geranium has a refreshing, antidepressant quality, good for nervous tension and exhaustion.

YLANG YLANG (*CANANGA ODORATA* VAR. *GENUINA*)

This tropical tree, native to Indonesia, produces an intensely sweet essential oil that has a sedative yet antidepressant action. It is good for many symptoms of excessive tension such as insomnia, panic attacks, anxiety and depression. It also has a good reputation as an aphrodisiac, through its ability to reduce stress levels.

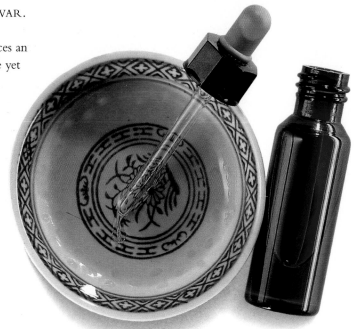

PEPPERMINT (*MENTHA PIPERITA*)

This oil is another classic ingredient in inhalations for relieving catarrh, although commercially menthol (a major part of the oil) may be used. Peppermint's analgesic and antispasmodic effects make it very useful for rubbing on to the temples to ease tension headaches; ideally dilute a drop in a little base cream or oil before applying.

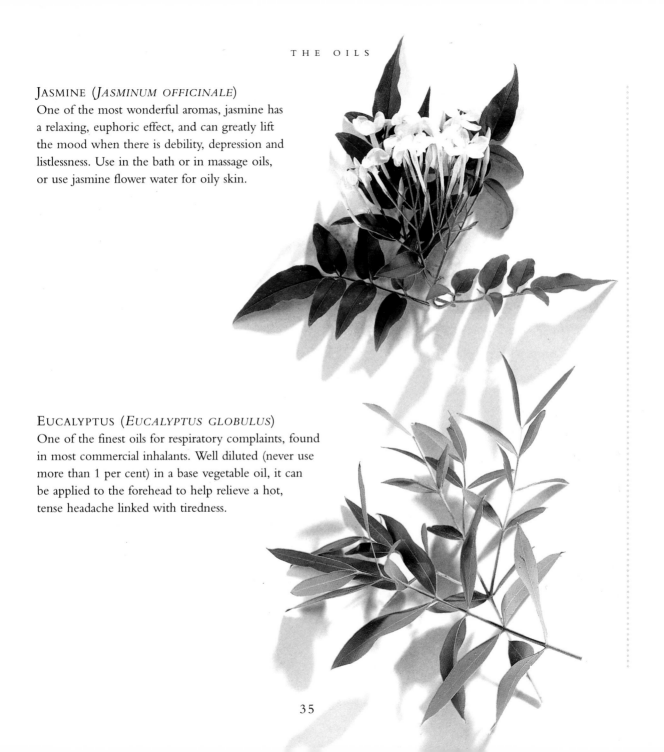

JASMINE (*JASMINUM OFFICINALE*)

One of the most wonderful aromas, jasmine has
a relaxing, euphoric effect, and can greatly lift
the mood when there is debility, depression and
listlessness. Use in the bath or in massage oils,
or use jasmine flower water for oily skin.

EUCALYPTUS (*EUCALYPTUS GLOBULUS*)

One of the finest oils for respiratory complaints, found
in most commercial inhalants. Well diluted (never use
more than 1 per cent) in a base vegetable oil, it can
be applied to the forehead to help relieve a hot,
tense headache linked with tiredness.

35

LAVENDER (*LAVANDULA ANGUSTIFOLIA*)

One of the most well-known scents, lavender has been used for centuries to refresh and add fragrance to the home, and as a remedy for stress-related ailments. It is especially helpful for tension headaches, or for nervous digestive upsets; use in a massage oil or in the bath for a deeply relaxing and calming experience.

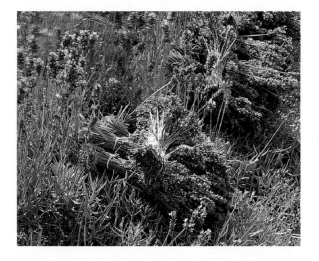

The finest oil is produced from the true lavender (*Lavandula angustifolia*), and is one of the safest and most versatile of all oils. Its uses range from first-aid treatment of burns, to skin care products, oils for muscular aches and pains, smelling salts for shock, and a host of stress-reducing applications.

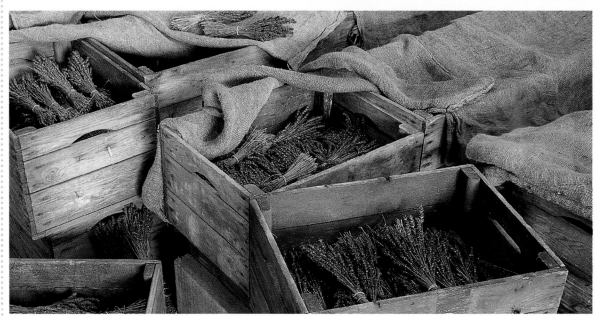

Lavender used to be grown extensively in England, but today France and Spain are the principal producers.

ROSEMARY (*ROSMARINUS OFFICINALIS*)

With a very penetrating, stimulating aroma, rosemary has been used for centuries to help to relieve nervous exhaustion, tension headaches and migraines. It improves circulation to the brain, and is an excellent oil for mental fatigue and debility.

MARJORAM (*ORIGANUM MARJORANA*)

Marjoram has a calming and warming effect, and is good for both cold, tight muscles and for cold, tense people who might suffer from headaches, migraines and insomnia. Use in massage blends for rubbing into tired and aching muscles, or in the bath, especially in the evening to help to obtain a good night's sleep.

PINE (*PINUS SYLVESTRIS*)

There are a few species of pine that produce oils, notably the American long-leaf pine which is a commercial source of oil of turpentine. However, the pine oil used in aromatherapy generally comes from the Scots pine. It helps to clear the air passages when used as an inhalation, and is also good for relieving fatigue. Tired, aching muscles can be eased with massage using diluted pine oil.

CLARY SAGE (*SALVIA SCLAREA*)

This oil gives a definite euphoric uplift to the brain; do not use too much, however, as you can be left feeling very spacey! Like ylang ylang and jasmine, its antidepressant and relaxing qualities have contributed to its reputation as an aphrodisiac.

ROSE *(ROSA X DAMASCENA, CENTIFOLIA)*

Rose is probably the most famous of all oils, prized since the beginning of time both as a marvellous fragrance and as a valuable remedy for many ailments. There is probably more symbolism attached to roses than any other flower, and their scent can evoke a general sense of pleasure and happiness.

Several kinds of roses have been used to extract the oil, notably the damask rose and the cabbage rose. Each one is slightly different, but the overall actions are sedating, calming and anti-inflammatory. Not surprisingly, rose oil has a wide reputation as an aphrodisiac, and where anxiety is a factor, it may be very beneficial. Use in the bath for a sensual, unwinding experience, or add to a base massage oil to soothe muscular and nervous tension.

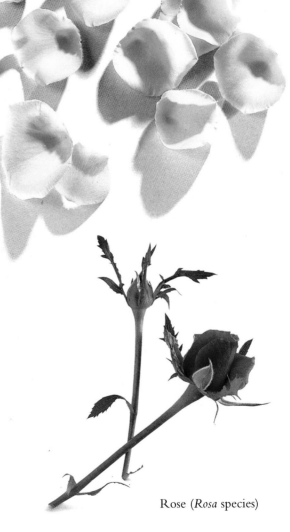

Rose (*Rosa* species)

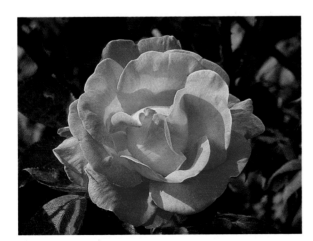

CITRUS OILS

Many citrus fruits yield essential oils, and they tend to have similar properties. In general they are refreshing, stimulating oils, good for the morning bath, leaving you feeling cleansed and alive.

BERGAMOT (*CITRUS BERGAMIA*)

The peel of the ripe fruit yields an oil that is mild and gentle. It is the most effective antidepressant oil of all, best used at the start of the day. Its leaves give the distinctive aroma and flavour to Earl Grey tea. The oil can be used on a burner for generally lifting the atmosphere. Do not use on the skin in bright sunlight, as it increases photosensitivity.

BITTER ORANGE (*CITRUS AURANTIUM* VAR. *AMARA*)

The bitter, or Seville, orange is the source of not one but three different oils, from the fruit, the blossom (also called neroli) and the leaf (also called petitgrain). These have overlapping effects; neroli is especially good as a tonic and mood lifter, raising the spirits and maybe the libido.

LEMON (*CITRUS LIMON*)

Possibly the most cleansing and antiseptic of the citrus oils, useful for boosting the immune system and in skin care. It can also refresh and clarify thoughts.

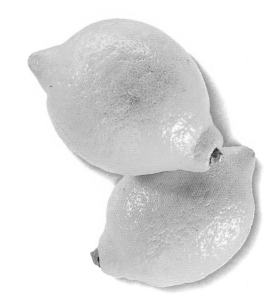

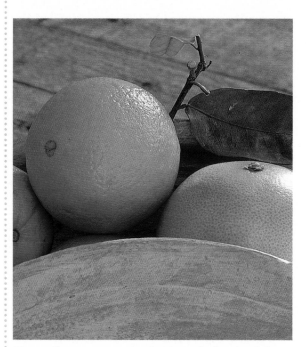

Citrus oils are great tonics, having a fresh, stimulating aroma to lift the mood and spirits.

MANDARIN (*CITRUS RETICULATA*)

Refreshing and cleansing, this sweetly scented oil is especially good for skin problems such as acne. It also helps digestion, soothing heartburn and nausea.

GRAPEFRUIT (*CITRUS X PARADISI*)

Oil of grapefruit is very helpful in the digestion of fatty foods and helps to combat cellulite and congested pores. It has an uplifting effect and will soothe headaches and nervous exhaustion.

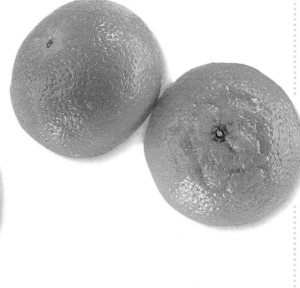

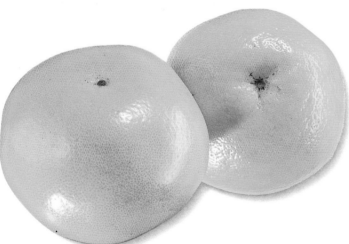

LIMES *(CITRUS AURANTIFOLIA)*

Oil of lime is good for stimulating a sluggish system and may be used when a tonic is needed, in massage or in the bath.

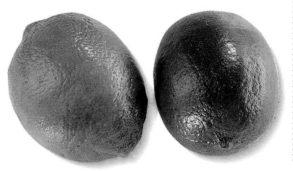

THERAPEUTIC RECIPES:

ONE OF THE DELIGHTS of aromatherapy is the blending together of oils for an enhanced therapeutic effect, with a new fragrance to soothe the senses at the same time. On the following pages you will find ideas for using combinations of oils; these have been created for their healing properties, but they also combine well in aroma. The sense of smell is very individual, so if you do not like a particular combination, try making your own blends, bearing in mind the actions of the oils and the dilution rates described earlier.

Try to ensure you buy good quality essential oils, with a pure scent that comes from the natural, unadulterated extract. Let your nose tell you of the quality and if a blend is harmonious, but above all if you enjoy the aroma.

For each of the blends suggested in this section, the number of drops of oils given should be diluted for massage purposes in 20 ml (4 tsp) of a base vegetable oil such as sweet almond oil. For a steam inhalation, use the number of drops given in a large bowl holding about 1 litre (1¾ pints) of hot water, and for a compress add the specified number of oil drops to a bowl holding 250 ml (8 fl oz) of hot water.

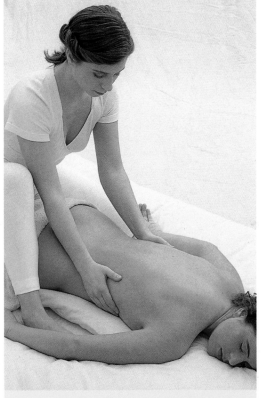

Taking time to relax and unwind with an aromatherapy massage is a wonderful and natural way to ease the body of stored tensions.

Right: Using essential oils in your daily routine is not only pleasurable but is also a means of improving your health and vitality.

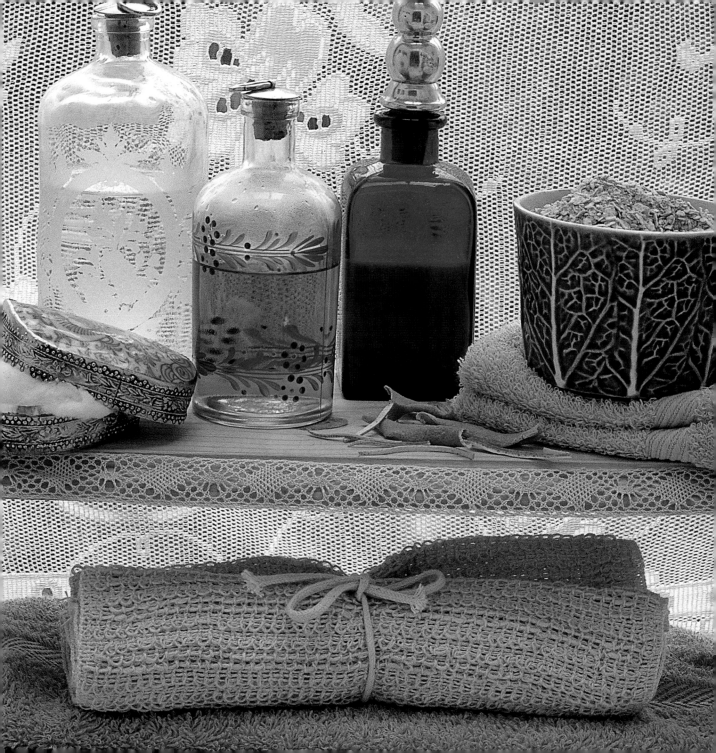

ANXIETY CALMERS

When people are described as being "uptight", that is often exactly what they are: tense muscles in the face and neck are a sure sign of anxiety. Release that tension with a face massage, using gentle, soothing strokes on the temples and forehead especially. This is very good as an evening treat, calming away the day's cares and worries.

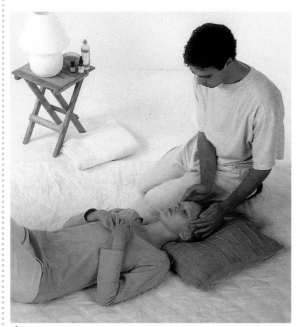

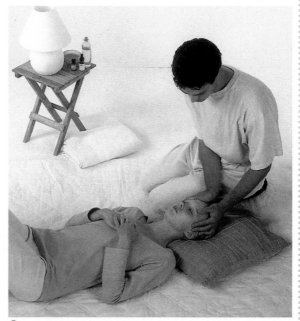

1 Ideally have the person lying down with the head in your lap or on a cushion. With your fingertips, gently smooth the essential oil blend into the face and head to aid relaxation.

Use just a little oil, as most people do not like a greasy feeling on the face. Make up a blend of 4 drops lavender and 2 drops ylang ylang in a light oil such as sweet almond, grapeseed or coconut.

2 Using your thumbs one after the other, stroke tension away from the centre of the forehead.

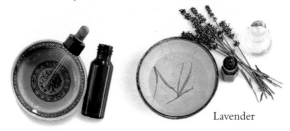

Lavender

BACKACHE RELIEVERS

So often people carry around their tensions in the form of a stiff, aching or knotted back. Symptoms can range from tight shoulders to lower backache, and the best way of using the essential oils is in massage of the taut muscles. Use long, sweeping strokes and a deeper kneading action to loosen areas of spasm, and let the aromatic oils work their magic at the same time.

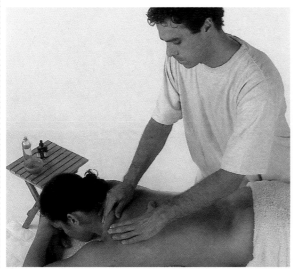

1 Knead the shoulders to ease stiff muscles.

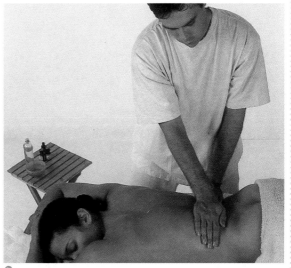

2 Apply steady, sweeping movements with the hands.

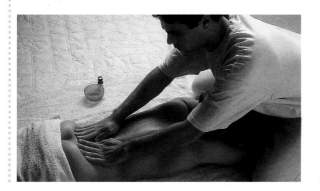

◄ 3 Stroke firmly down the back with both hands.

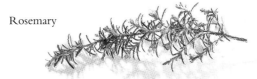

Rosemary

Two essential oil blends that will help to work on the deeper tensions and knotted muscles are 3 drops pine and 3 drops rosemary, or 4 drops lavender and 3 drops marjoram mixed with the base oil.

UPLIFTING OILS

There are unfortunately times in all our lives when we get depressed to some extent, whether due to a specific event or from chronic tiredness. As part of a programme of recuperation and restoring vitality, aromatherapy can be very effective in lifting the mood and overall energy.

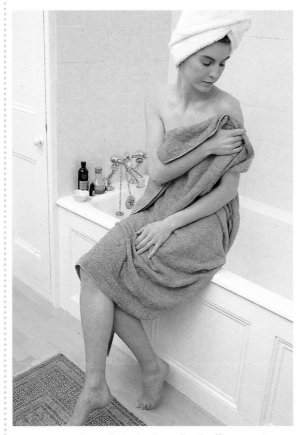

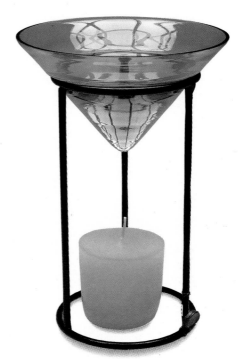

A gentler effect, which can pervade the atmosphere all day long, is to use bergamot or neroli oils in an essential oil burner – probably just one drop of each oil at a time, repeating as needed.

For a strong, but relatively short-lived effect, try 4 drops bergamot and 2 drops neroli in the bath, ideally in the morning. After the bath, gently pat the skin with a soft towel. Do not rub vigorously.

SKIN TONICS

When we become stressed, the small muscles close to the skin tend to contract. This can leave our skin under-nourished with blood, and over time our complexion and skin tone suffer. Apart from dealing with the underlying worries, the skin itself can also be helped with essential oils. Tense skin is frequently drier than normal, and probably the best way to use the oils is to mix them into your favourite skin cream. Obviously this is best if the cream is originally unperfumed.

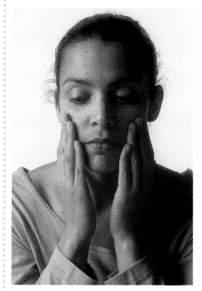

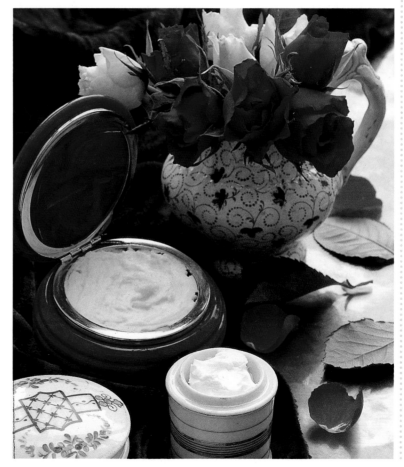

Above: To a 25 g (1oz) pot of skin cream, add either 3 drops rose and 3 drops sandalwood, or 4 drops neroli and 2 drops rose and apply to the skin.

Right: As with all essential oil blends, it is best if you only mix up small amounts of cream and oil at a time.

HEADACHE EASERS

Tension headaches are a common feature in many people's lives, and may come from long hours at the computer or even longer hours with small children! Whatever the cause, gentle massage of the temples and forehead at the earliest moment can help to stop headaches from getting a tight grip. Another option is a warm compress.

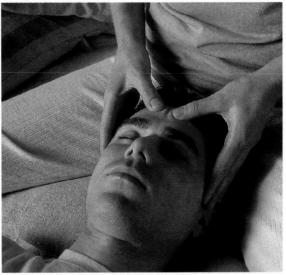

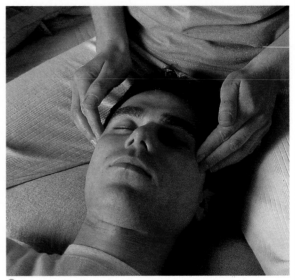

1 Ease tension headaches by massaging oils into the forehead. With your thumbs, use steady but gentle pressure to stroke the forehead.

2 Gently massage the temples with the fingers to release tension and stress.

• If the head feels hot, try using an oil with 4 drops peppermint.
• If warmth feels as though it is helpful, use 6 drops lavender.
• Another option for either type of headache is 4 drops chamomile.

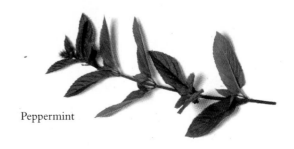

Peppermint

HIGH BLOOD PRESSURE RELIEVER

It should be emphasized that anyone with very high blood pressure should first seek medical (or professional) treatment. In milder cases, related to anxiety and tension, you can help to get temporary relief by using essential oils. A very good way to do so is in a footbath, the warmth from the water helping to bring blood to the feet and reduce the blood pressure.

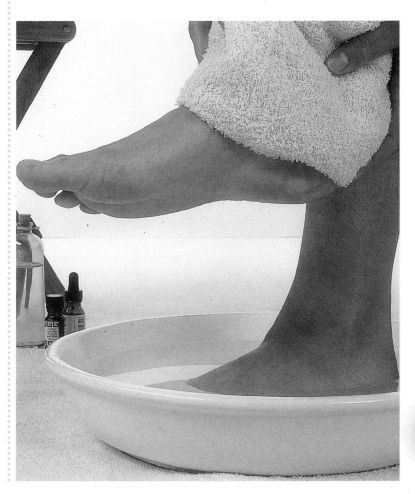

Fill a large bowl three-quarters full with hot water and add 2 drops rose, 2 drops ylang ylang and 3 drops lavender.

Carefully let the feet sink into the water and soak for at least 5 minutes.

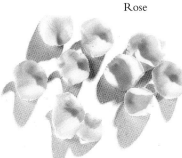

Rose

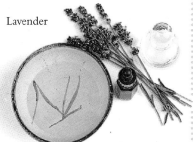

Lavender

SLEEP ENHANCERS

Worries can go round and round inside our heads, usually just as we are trying to get to sleep. The resulting disturbed and restless night leaves us more prone to stress and anxiety, and a vicious cycle can be created. Help break into this cycle with a pleasantly hot and relaxing evening bath. Many oils can be useful – just having a fragrance that you enjoy will help you to unwind after a long day.

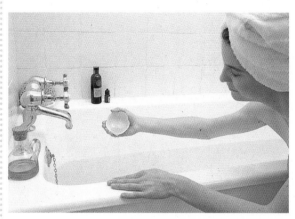

Above: Add oils to an evening bath to aid relaxation and sleep. A couple of relaxing blends, without over-sedating, are 4 drops rose and 3 drops sandalwood or 5 drops lavender and 3 drops ylang ylang.

Right: Incorporate aromatherapy preparations into your daily bathing routine.

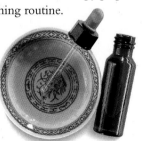

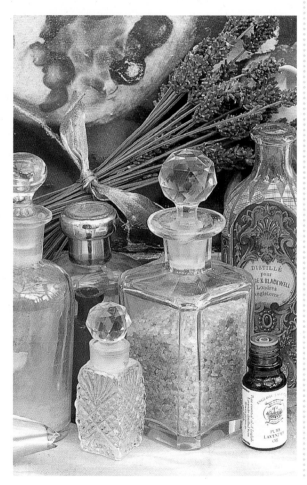

DIGESTIVE SETTLERS

Nervousness often shows itself in an upset stomach, or abdominal spasms. It has been said that our digestive organs also digest stress, and too often they end up storing emotions, causing all manner of discomfort and indigestion. The key is to allow our bodies to let go of such worries and anxieties, and aromatherapy can help a great deal to achieve this. One of the easiest ways to use oils in this context is to make a hot compress and place it over the abdomen, keeping the area warm for up to 10 minutes.

Use a bowl of hot water, with either 2 drops orange and 3 drops peppermint or 3 drops chamomile and 2 drops orange.

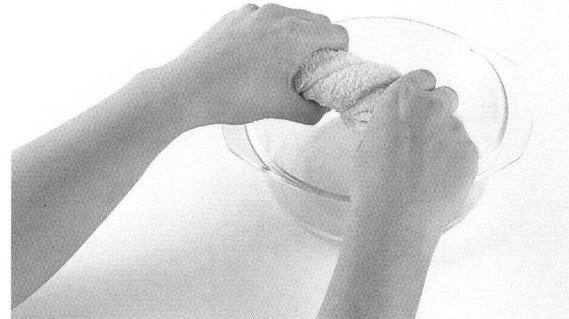

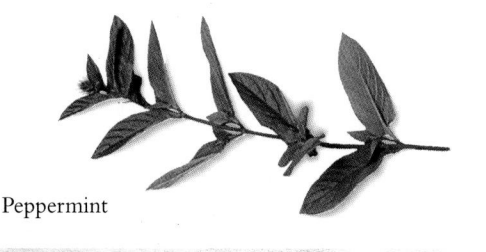

Peppermint

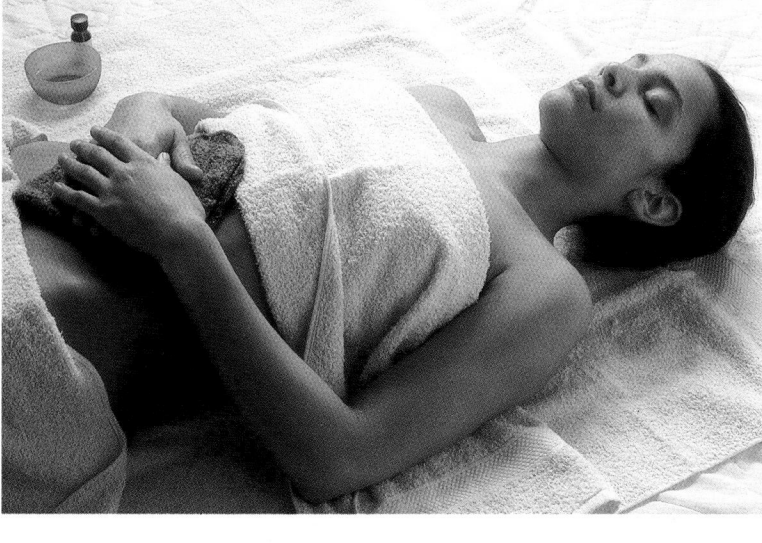

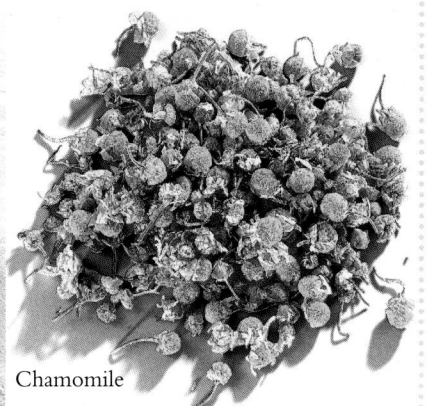

Chamomile

Above: Soak a flannel in a bowl of hot water. Left: Place the compress over the abdomen and relax.

TRAVEL CALMERS

They say that travel broadens the mind; unfortunately, for some people it contracts the mind into a series of worries – will the car break down? Is this plane safe? Will I be sick? If you are a poor or anxious traveller, try using one of the following essential oils to calm the mind and stomach, letting you enjoy the delights of new horizons without being stressed by how to reach them.

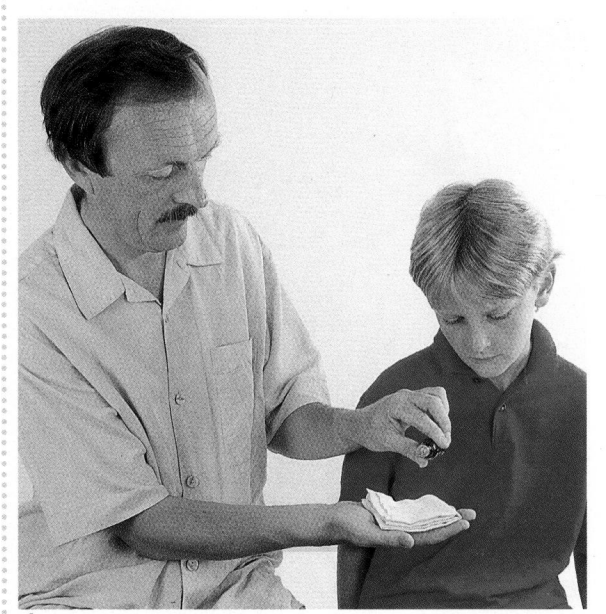

1 Put a couple of drops of essential oil on a tissue.

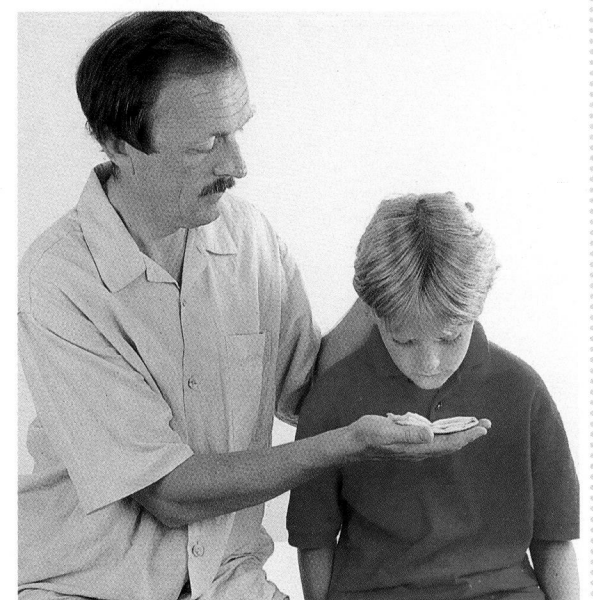

2 Hold the tissue under the nose and lean the head slightly forward. Inhale.

The simplest way to use essential oils when travelling is to put a couple of drops on to a tissue or handkerchief, and smell them frequently. Useful oils are peppermint, mandarin or neroli.

Peppermint

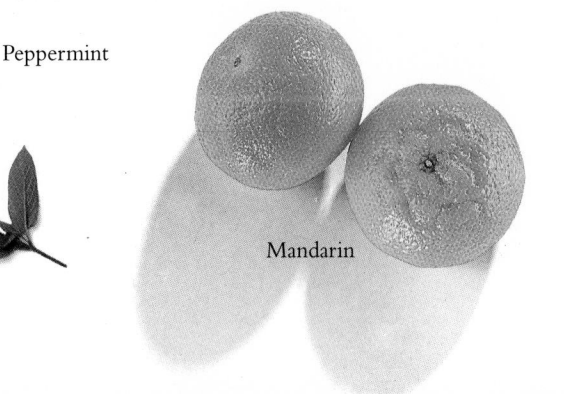

Mandarin

PRE-MENSTRUAL TENSION SOOTHERS

For many women the days leading up to a period can be fraught with mood swings, irritability and other symptoms. Professional treatment may be needed for full assistance; however, try this blend of oils if before each period you feel very tense and critical of those around you, or just want to devour a box of chocolates!

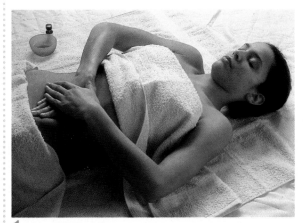

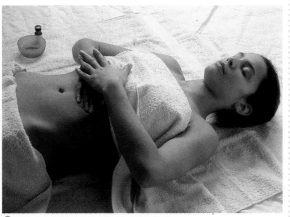

1 Slowly and firmly massage the abdomen with your hands.

2 Move your hands in a clockwise direction; try to remain relaxed the whole time.

Either add 3 drops rose, 3 drops jasmine and 2 drops clary sage to a bath and lie back allowing the tension to soak away, or use this mixture in a massage oil and rub gently into the abdomen for a relaxing, soothing effect.

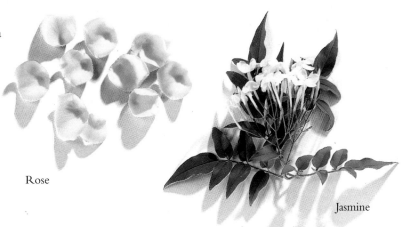

Rose

Jasmine

MIGRAINE EASERS

One of the most complex of health problems, migraines are nature's way of shutting us down when life has been too demanding. The triggers that spark off a migraine attack are highly individual and professional treatment is really needed to try to understand the causes for each person. Many migraine sufferers have a heightened sense of smell at the onset of the attack and may find any aroma intolerable, so use oils sparingly and carefully.

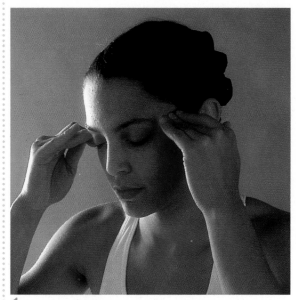

1 For self-help, gently massage the temples with small circling movements.

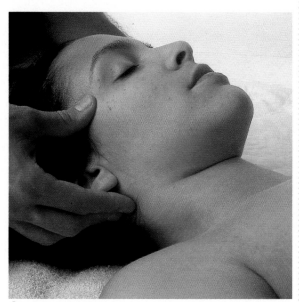

2 A gentle head massage from a partner can be even more beneficial.

At the earliest stage of a migraine, try using a blend of 2 drops rosemary, 1 drop marjoram and 1 drop clary sage, diluted in a massage oil and very gently massaged into the temples and forehead. Alternatively, use a drop of each oil in a bowl of warm water and apply a compress to the forehead.

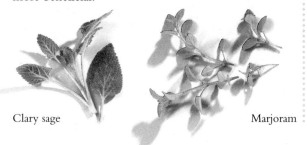

Clary sage   Marjoram

MILD SHOCK SOOTHERS

You bump your head, trip over the cat, fall down the stairs, get the gas bill . . . we all have times when we get rather shaken up and suffer from mild shock. We may feel a little dizzy or faint, and need to sit down. At these times, essential oils can be a useful first-aid help, bringing us back to our senses.

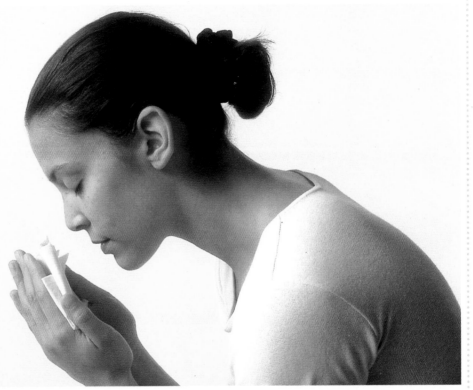

The quickest and simplest way to benefit from aromatherapy in instances of mild shock is to put an open bottle of either lavender or clary sage oil under the person's nose and let them sniff the aroma directly. Otherwise, put a couple of oil drops on a tissue, hold under the nose and inhale.

CAUTION:
Remember, never try to treat a case of severe shock at home. Seek medical advice immediately.

MUSCULAR ACHE RELIEVERS

When you are under stress for any length of time, your body stays permanently tense. This can make any or all of your muscles ache and feel tired or heavy. To relieve these symptoms, and also to begin to release the underlying tension, use essential oils in a massage blend. As the massage movements work on the aching muscles, the oils are being absorbed and get to work on inner tension too.

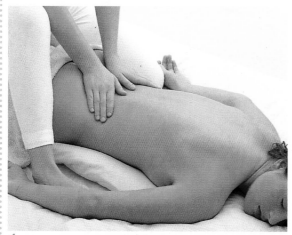

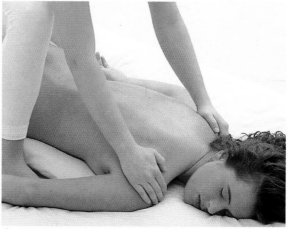

1 Rest your hands on the lower back either side of the spine. Lean your weight into your hands and stroke firmly up the back towards the head. Mould your hands to the body as they glide along.

2 As your hands reach the top of the back, fan them out towards the shoulders in a flowing motion.

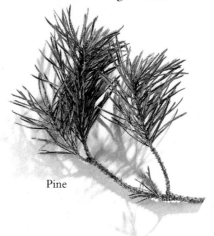

Pine

Marjoram

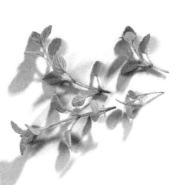

Use a blend of 3 drops pine, 3 drops marjoram and 2 drops juniper for a variety of soothing massage strokes.

REVITALIZING OILS

In today's high pressure world, trying to juggle with too many demands leads nearly all of us to reach a state of "brain fag" at some point, when mental fatigue and exhaustion grind us to a halt. Rather than reach for the coffee, or worse still alcohol, which may seem to relax but actually depresses the central nervous system, try using these revitalizing oils to give you an instant pick-me-up and make you feel more alert.

Below: You can use 1–2 drops of rosemary or peppermint oil in a burner. Alternatively, add 3 drops rosemary and 2 drops peppermint to a bowl of steaming water, or use 4 drops of either oils on their own. Allow the oils to evaporate into the room and breathe freely.

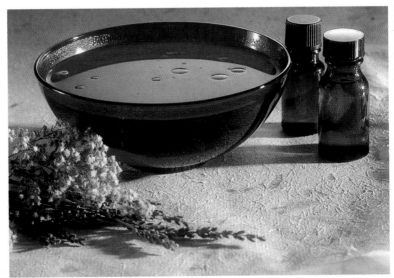

Vaporized essential oils are invaluable for balancing the emotions.

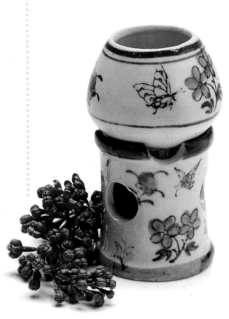

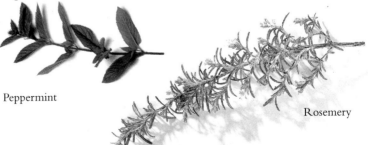

Peppermint

Rosemery

STRESS RELIEVERS

Stress, or rather our inability to cope with an excess amount of it, is one of the biggest health problems today. Lifestyles seem to include so many demands that it is not surprising that most of us feel stressed at times, sometimes constantly. We all react to excessive stress in different ways, with tension, anxiety, depression or exhaustion, but we can all benefit from the wonderfully balancing and stress-busting effects of aromatic oils.

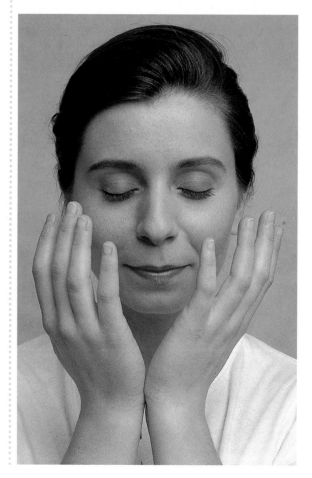

Our bodies are geared to cope with a stressful situation by producing various hormones that trigger off a series of physiological actions in the body; these are known collectively as the "fight or flight" syndrome, and serve to place the body in a state of alert in a potentially dangerous situation. Extra blood is shunted to the muscles, and the heart rate speeds up while the digestion slows down. These responses are appropriate when we are faced with a physical threat, but can nowadays be triggered by quite different kinds of stress and end up placing a strain on our bodies without fulfilling any useful need.

In order to help reduce the impact of stress on the whole system, it is necessary to find ways both to avoid getting over-stressed in the first instance and to let go of the changes that occur internally under stress. Aromatherapy can help in each case, the oils helping to keep you calm under pressure and releasing inner tensions following stress, especially in massage.

To prevent undue stress, try simply inhaling one of your favourite oils at regular intervals, or put a couple of drops in a burner in your room or office, to help keep you feeling more relaxed and calm.

Left: It should not take you long to discover which essential oils work best for you as an individual.

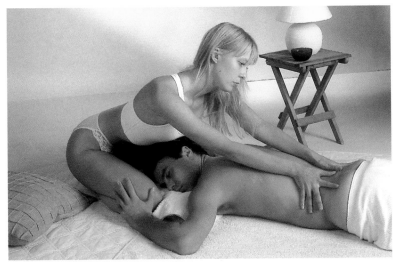

If possible, use one of the following blends in a base oil, and get your partner to massage you for the perfect antidote to that overdose of life's stresses.

• For aiding relaxation, 3 drops lavender, 3 drops geranium and 3 drops marjoram.

• For both calming and soothing, as well as giving a gentle uplift, 4 drops rose and 3 drops jasmine.

• For a more definitely uplifting and energizing effect, try 3 drops clary sage and 4 drops bergamot.

1 Slowly and gently massage in the oil, moving your hands down each side of the spine.

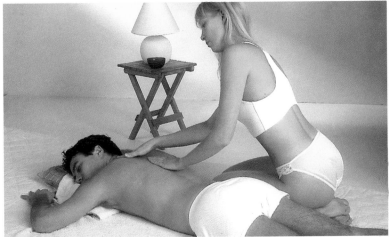

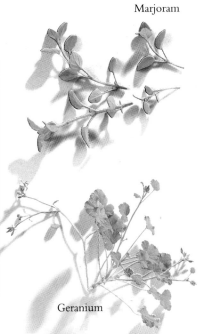

Marjoram

Geranium

2 For relaxation, use one hand after the other to stroke down the back in a steady rhythm.

SENSUAL OILS

Tension, anxiety, worry, depression – all these can affect your sexual energy and performance.
Sometimes this leads into a negative spiral of anxiety about sex leading to less enjoyment and
so on. Take a little time out of your hectic life to be together with your partner and have fun;
add to your sensual pleasure with an intimate massage session, using one of these blends to release
tensions and allow your natural sexual energy to respond.

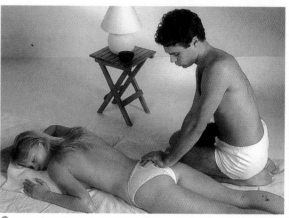

2 You can apply a firmer pressure over large muscles
such as the buttocks.

Use whichever of these blends – 5 drops rose and
5 drops sandalwood or 4 drops jasmine and 4 drops
ylang ylang – appeals to you both, and include in a
massage oil. Use gentle, stroking movements all over
the back, buttocks, legs and front.

Sandalwood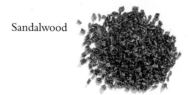

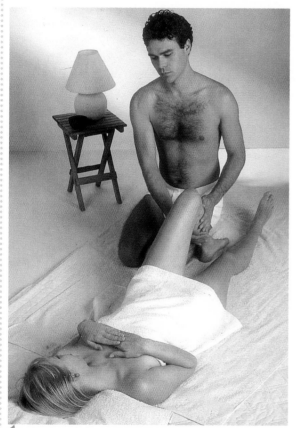

1 Massage gently all over the body with a light,
caring touch.

MENSTRUAL PAIN RELIEVERS

Painful periods can be due to a number of reasons, but tension will certainly add to muscle spasm and cramping pains. If there is no organic or structural cause of the discomfort, try using essential oils, either as a hot compress over the lower abdomen or in the bath. Some oils have a reputation for improving the menstrual cycle in other ways; seek advice from a professional aromatherapist for longer-term treatments.

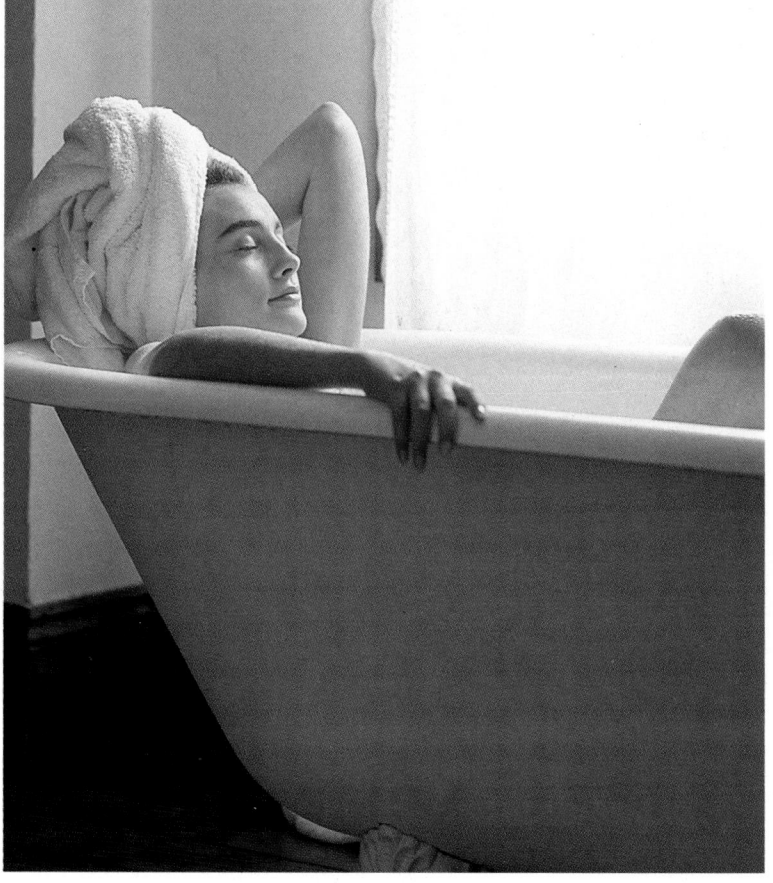

For a compress, use 1 drop of rose, geranium and clary sage oils. Alternatively, a fairly hot bath with 3 drops rose, 3 drops geranium and 2 drops clary sage will quickly relax cramped muscles.

Left: A long bath with a few drops of oil will help you to relax and to soothe away any discomfort.

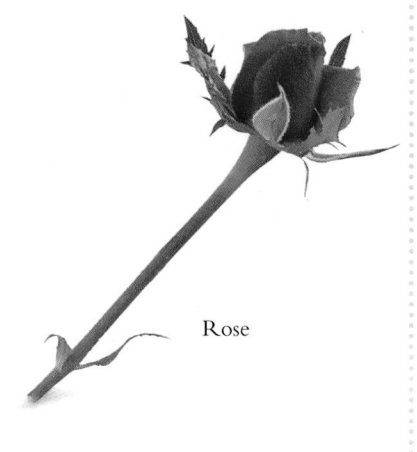

Rose

INVIGORATING OILS

Chronic tension all too often leads to a feeling of exhaustion, when we just run out of steam. At these times we need a boost, and many oils have a tonic effect, restoring vitality without over-stimulating. As a group, the citrus oils are good for this purpose, ranging from the more soothing mandarin to the very refreshing lemon oil.

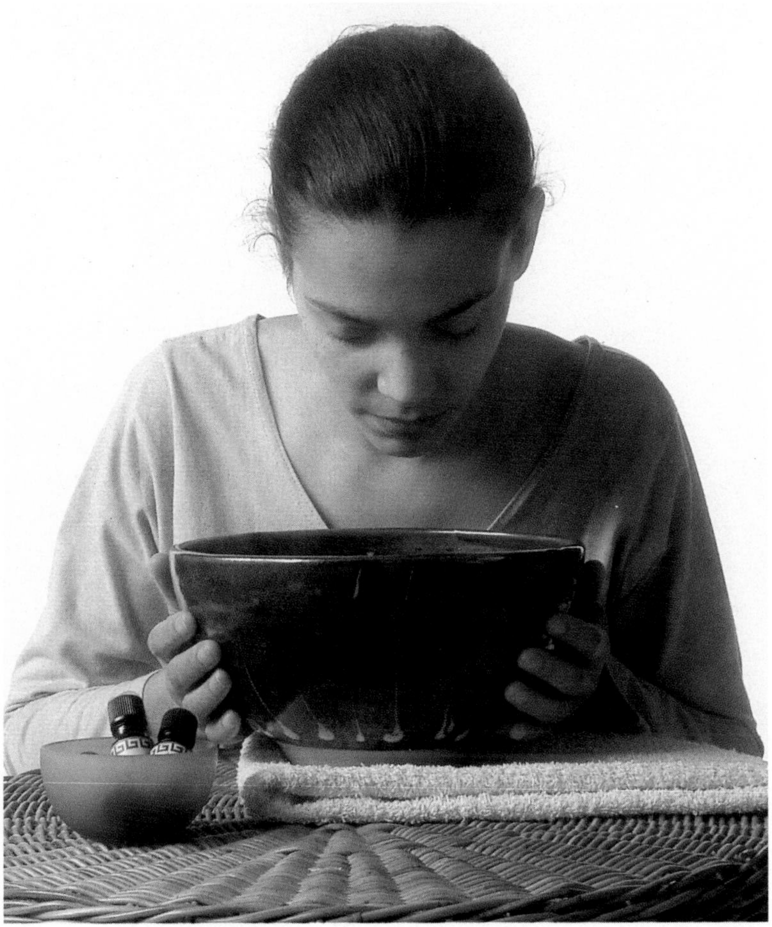

Have a warm, but not too hot bath, with 4 drops mandarin and 2 drops orange or 4 drops neroli and 2 drops lemon. Alternatively, just add a couple of drops of any of these oils to a bowl of steaming water and gently inhale to help to clear away the tiredness and lift your spirits.

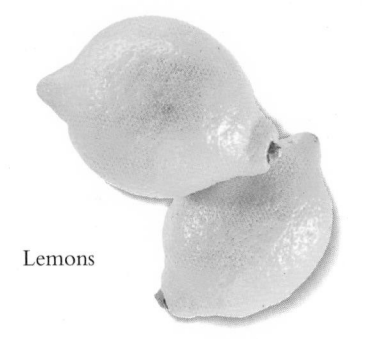

Lemons

Left: Steam inhalation is a valuable and simple way to receive the benefits of essential oils when time or circumstance prevent massage or a bath.

BREATHING ENHANCERS

"Breathe" . . . how often have we said this to ourselves when we are tense and stressed?
Although breathing occurs normally without our conscious control, it can be affected to a
considerable extent as we tense up, tightening the chest muscles and restricting lung expansion.

If you tend to tighten across the
chest, try using this aromatic blend
as a steam inhalation. To a bowl
of steaming water add 3 drops
benzoin, 2 drops marjoram and
2 drops eucalyptus.

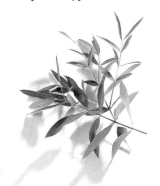

Eucalyptus

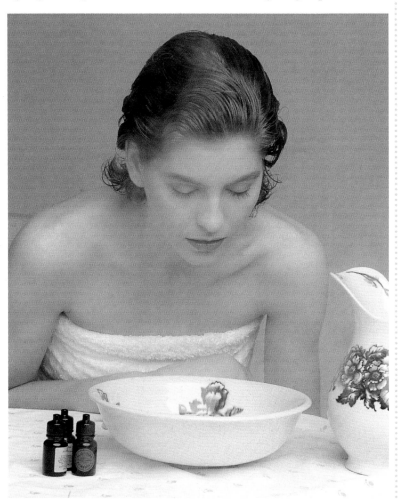

Right: As the oils vaporize, inhale
the steam deeply. If you hold a
towel over your head this will slow
down the evaporation.

INDEX

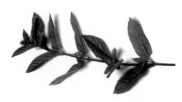

Photography credits: Don Last 3, 4, 6t, m, 11, 15, 17tl/tr, 18l, 19tr, 22–29, 31, 32tl/br, 33–35, 37, 38, 39t, 40r, 41, 44, 45, 48, 49l/tr, 50bl, 51, 53–55, 56bl, 57r, 59, 60, 61b, 62b/tl, 63l, 64t; Alistair Hughes pp 5b, 10, 12, 13, 14, 17bl, 21, 42, 46, 50tl, 52l, 56t, 57l, 58, 63r; John Freeman and Michelle Garrett p 2; Michelle Garrett pp 9, 16, 18r, 30, 40l, 43, 47r; Debbie Patterson pp 6, 7 14, 19l/b, 36, 50r and Lucy Mason pp 8, 20, 32bl, 39bl/br, 49br, 52r, 61t, 62tr, 64r.
t=top, b=bottom, l=left, r=right, m=middle.

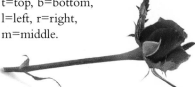

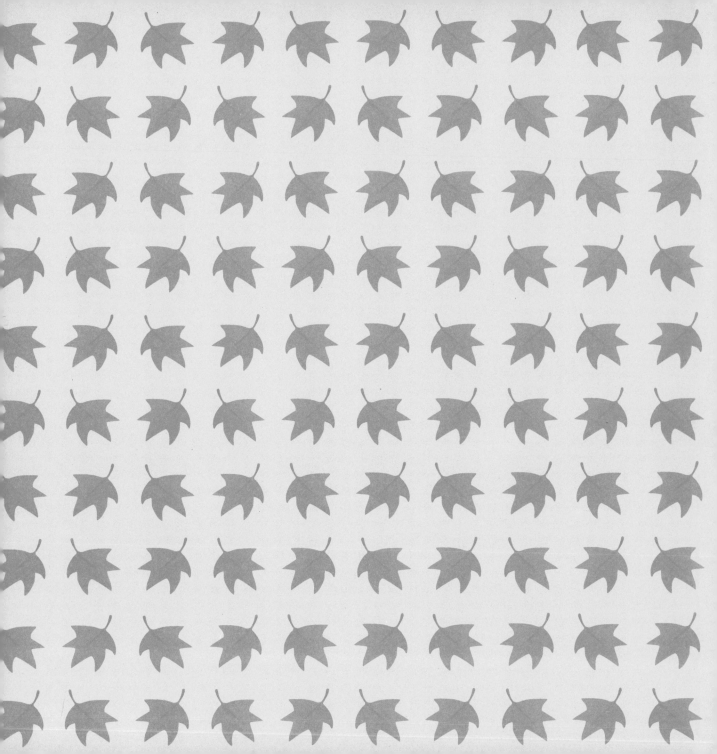